Seasonable thoughts and advices upon inoculation. In which (first) the benefits and advantages of that ... practice are set forth and illustrated. And by which (secondly) they are recommended ... By Dr. Perry.

Charles Perry

ECCO
PRINT EDITIONS

Seasonable thoughts and advices upon inoculation. In which (first) the benefits and advantages of that ... practice are set forth and illustrated. And by which (secondly) they are recommended ... By Dr. Perry.
Perry, Charles
ESTCID: N021566
Reproduction from National Library of Medicine
With a final errata leaf.
[London?] : Printed in the year, 1752.
58,[2]p. ; 8°

ECCO

Eighteenth Century Collections Online Print Editions

Gale ECCO Print Editions

Relive history with *Eighteenth Century Collections Online*, now available in print for the independent historian and collector. This series includes the most significant English-language and foreign-language works printed in Great Britain during the eighteenth century, and is organized in seven different subject areas including literature and language; medicine, science, and technology; and religion and philosophy. The collection also includes thousands of important works from the Americas.

The eighteenth century has been called "The Age of Enlightenment." It was a period of rapid advance in print culture and publishing, in world exploration, and in the rapid growth of science and technology – all of which had a profound impact on the political and cultural landscape. At the end of the century the American Revolution, French Revolution and Industrial Revolution, perhaps three of the most significant events in modern history, set in motion developments that eventually dominated world political, economic, and social life.

In a groundbreaking effort, Gale initiated a revolution of its own: digitization of epic proportions to preserve these invaluable works in the largest online archive of its kind. Contributions from major world libraries constitute over 175,000 original printed works. Scanned images of the actual pages, rather than transcriptions, recreate the works ***as they first appeared.***

Now for the first time, these high-quality digital scans of original works are available via print-on-demand, making them readily accessible to libraries, students, independent scholars, and readers of all ages.

For our initial release we have created seven robust collections to form one the world's most comprehensive catalogs of 18th century works.

Initial Gale ECCO Print Editions collections include:

History and Geography

Rich in titles on English life and social history, this collection spans the world as it was known to eighteenth-century historians and explorers. Titles include a wealth of travel accounts and diaries, histories of nations from throughout the world, and maps and charts of a world that was still being discovered. Students of the War of American Independence will find fascinating accounts from the British side of conflict.

Social Science
Delve into what it was like to live during the eighteenth century by reading the first-hand accounts of everyday people, including city dwellers and farmers, businessmen and bankers, artisans and merchants, artists and their patrons, politicians and their constituents. Original texts make the American, French, and Industrial revolutions vividly contemporary.

Medicine, Science and Technology
Medical theory and practice of the 1700s developed rapidly, as is evidenced by the extensive collection, which includes descriptions of diseases, their conditions, and treatments. Books on science and technology, agriculture, military technology, natural philosophy, even cookbooks, are all contained here.

Literature and Language
Western literary study flows out of eighteenth-century works by Alexander Pope, Daniel Defoe, Henry Fielding, Frances Burney, Denis Diderot, Johann Gottfried Herder, Johann Wolfgang von Goethe, and others. Experience the birth of the modern novel, or compare the development of language using dictionaries and grammar discourses.

Religion and Philosophy
The Age of Enlightenment profoundly enriched religious and philosophical understanding and continues to influence present-day thinking. Works collected here include masterpieces by David Hume, Immanuel Kant, and Jean-Jacques Rousseau, as well as religious sermons and moral debates on the issues of the day, such as the slave trade. The Age of Reason saw conflict between Protestantism and Catholicism transformed into one between faith and logic -- a debate that continues in the twenty-first century.

Law and Reference
This collection reveals the history of English common law and Empire law in a vastly changing world of British expansion. Dominating the legal field is the *Commentaries of the Law of England* by Sir William Blackstone, which first appeared in 1765. Reference works such as almanacs and catalogues continue to educate us by revealing the day-to-day workings of society.

Fine Arts
The eighteenth-century fascination with Greek and Roman antiquity followed the systematic excavation of the ruins at Pompeii and Herculaneum in southern Italy; and after 1750 a neoclassical style dominated all artistic fields. The titles here trace developments in mostly English-language works on painting, sculpture, architecture, music, theater, and other disciplines. Instructional works on musical instruments, catalogs of art objects, comic operas, and more are also included.

SEASONABLE THOUGHTS
AND
ADVICES
UPON
INOCULATION.

IN WHICH

(*Firſt*) the Benefits and Advantages of that moſt rational and ſalutary Practice are ſet forth and illuſtrated.

AND BY WHICH

(*Secondly*) they are recommended to the Publick (at this Time more eſpecially) in order to encourage and promote it.

By Dr. PERRY.

Printed in the Year MDCCLII.

SEASONABLE

THOUGHTS and ADVICES

UPON

INOCULATION.

THOUGH the Practice of Inoculating the Small Pox is what I have long approv'd, and strenuously recommended—yet the present Crisis (when the Distemper has not only got Footing in the Capital of the County, but in many circumjacent Towns and Villages also) more especially excites my Desires and Endeavours to encourage and promote so rational and salutary a Practice as much as possible.——To this End, and to this Purpose, I will consider the said Subject on every Side; and in every Light, perhaps, that it will admit of.——And I hope to make appear, plainly and clearly, that the Practice of Inoculation is consistent with Reason and Religion;—with good Sense and common Prudence.——And lastly, that it is, in some Measure, accessary and necessary to the Preservation of the human Kind;---as also to their Ease, Comfort and Happiness.

THIS Practice of inoculating the Small-Pox was, indeed, but of late Years introduced amongst us.—And it is not as yet an established Practice—but is only approv'd of and practised here and there—or by particular Parties and Setts of People.—Nevertheless it brought with it from *Turkey* (the Country whence we received it) a high Sanction and Authority.—For though the *Turks* seldom practice it amongst themselves—being rigid *Predestinarians*,——yet amongst the *Arminians*, the *Georgians*, the *Mingretians*, and the *Circassians*, as also amongst the *Greeks*, it has been in general Use from Time immemorial;—which may be admitted as a presumptive Proof of its Expediency and Usefulness.

I KNOW very well that many Pieces (*pro* and *con.*) have been penn'd and publish'd upon this Subject,——most of which I have read;——but as these are now out of my Hands, and almost forgot by me, so I will leave them entirely out of the Question, and proceed to deliver my own private Sentiments upon the Matter.

As to the Specific Opperation call'd Inoculation,—I never had (I own it) any Experience or Concern in it.—For as I never had the Small-Pox——so I never perform'd the Opperation of Inoculating——nor so much as assisted in it.——Otherwise, from the many Debates and Conversations which I have had upon that Subject (during my Travels) with Persons perfectly well versed and practised in it, I might presume to assert myself as well qualified to undertake it as any Person in the Realm. However, the Business of Inoculating (which is very easy in itself) is well understood by many Persons,—and is pretty well guessed at by myself. And it is with no small Pleasure I observe, that the

the Wiſdom and Prudence of the People in many Parts of the Nation, have led them readily to embrace and practice it:—But what more eſpecially gives me Pleaſure and Satisfaction at this preſent Time, is to hear, that ſeveral Perſons hereabout intend ſpeedily to be inoculated;—and particularly that Mr. *Paul*, an eminent Surgeon at *Stroud*, has opened the Scene here—by inoculating his only Son and his Neice. I mention this Inſtance of Mr. *Paul*'s inoculating his Son and his Neice,—not only as a Tribute of Praiſe to his good Senſe, and Prudence, ſhewn in the Thing, but in Hopes alſo that it may inſtruct, influence, and induce all Perſons hereabouts who have not had the ſmall Pox, readily to embrace, and ſubmit to ſo eaſy, ſo ſafe, and ſo reaſonable a Practice.

I HAVE (as above ſaid) read ſeveral Pieces (*pro* and *con*) upon this Subject,—and I have been a Party in many Debates, and Controverſies upon the ſame Subject.——And when I ſum up all the Arguments on both Sides—as well ideal and ſpeculative, as real and written,——I find myſelf oblig'd to give my Voice and Vote in Favour of Inoculation. But tho' this laudable, ſalutary Practice of Inoculation is pretty generally approv'd of by all rational, conſiderate, unprejudiced Perſons,—yet (and I am ſorry that I have Room and Reaſon to ſay it) it is not quite univerſally ſubſcribed to,--even by Perſons of good Senſe, ſolid Reaſon, and ſober Reflection.——What therefore (to put a Queſtion) can this Diviſion, and Diſſention amongſt Mankind, upon ſo plain and obvious an Affair, proceed from? Why; (to make Anſwer to the ſuppoſed Queſtion) I plainly ſee that 'tis made a Party Affair, I mean of a religious Nature;—for the Diſ-

ſenters

ters, and others who go under the Diſtinction and Denomination of Whigs, almoſt univerſally approve it, and many of them practice it.—Whereas many of thoſe who are on the other Side of the Queſtion (in Religious Matters) diſapprove, and condemn it.—Nevertheleſs Inoculation will always (I'll vouch for it) ſupport its Credit and Reputation in the Opinions, Eſtimation, and Judgment of all reaſonable, diſpaſſionate, unprejudic'd Perſons.—And the Approbation and Preference it juſtly lays Claim to, will, I preſume, appear inconteſtable, from the following ſhort Eſtimate of Matters.

FIRST. It is univerſally maintain'd, and allow'd, that not above one Perſon in a Dozen lives to an advanced Age, without taking the Small Pox in the natural Way, unleſs it was eluded by Inoculation.—*Secondly.* By an accurate, impartial and faithful Eſtimate, it appears (on an Average) that about one ſixth Part generally die of the Small Pox, of ſuch as take it in the natural Way.—This is a juſt Eſtimate as Things happen at common Times—tho' at ſome particular Times, and in ſome particular Places, the Small Pox in the natural Way, is ſo mild and favourable that not above one in Ten or a Dozen dies of it.—Now let us look into the State of the Caſe—as it generally happens, and obtains under the Practice of Inoculation—it is poſitively aſſerted and maintained by the Advocates for Inoculation (and I muſt take it for Truth, as I never heard it denied, or even diſputed by the oppoſite Party) that at this Time not ſo much as one in an Hundred dies of the Small Pox by Inoculation—(though 'till within a few Years paſt the Eſtimate was not ſo much in its favour.) And hence it appears plain (cou'd no other Reasons against it, or Objections to it be exhibited) that Inoculation is by far the more easy, safe and eligible Way of proceeding.——But besides these visible and incontestable Advantages—should all Mankind embrace and practice this Method—every one doubtless wou'd have their Children, Relations, and Friends inoculated, within that Period of Life called Childhood—before they cou'd reasonably be suppos'd to have contracted any ill Habits, or Distemperatures in the Blood and Animal Juices.——And what would necessarily be the Consequence of this? Why, all those who had submitted to, and happily passed thro' this Operation——wou'd for the future be perfectly free of that Terror and Dread, which so continually haunt many Persons who never had this Distemper.——By this Method brought into general Use and Practice, the Small Pox wou'd soon be divested of its Dread and Terror; and wou'd be look'd upon as a mild, benign and favourable Visitor.

Before I proceed any further, 'tis both just and proper that I bring under my Inspection and Examination, the two grand and most important Objections to Inoculation.——And, (*First*) the Theologists (some of them at least) tell us, that the Practice of Inoculation is unchristian and impious.----That it is a tempting and provoking of God Almighty.——That it is the thwarting his Designs and Purposes.——That it is usurping upon God's Prerogative; and taking his proper Work (that of inflicting Diseases) out of his Hands.——But these Arguments and Objections (however specious and persuasive they may appear to some) are what, I fancy, the more rational, candid and

unpre-

unprejudiced Part of Mankind will ſcarcely ſubſcribe to.——The *Second* Objection brought againſt it (which is uſed by ſome minute Philoſophers; and perhaps, by ſome minute Phyſicians too) is this,—namely, That poſſibly—and perhaps ——and ſo forth——the latent inviſible Seeds, or Stamina, of ſome ill Habit, or chronical Diſeaſe (ſuch for Example, as the Scorbutic, the Scrofulous, the Strumous, the Cancerous, the Leprous, the Ganty, the Nephritic, and what not) might exiſt in the Blood of the Perſon from whom the inoculating Matter was taken;—and that the ſuppoſed latent inviſible Seeds may be transfuſed together with the variolous Matter, into the Habit or Blood of the Perſon Inoculated——And laſtly, that (thereafter) the ſuppoſed latent inviſible morbic Seeds, or Stamina, may vegetate fœcundate multiply and encreaſe,——ſo far as to produce and manifeſt the ſame corrupt vicious Habit, in the Subject Inoculated, as was inherent (tho' latent and concealed) in the Blood of the Perſon from whom the inoculating Matter was taken. Now, as concerning the firſt mentioned Objection, this is confeſſedly, a Thing rather preſumed than proved;----ſo with regard to that we may ſay, ——-*Adhuc ſubjudice lis eſt*. For we find that People of different Perſuaſions (tho' of the ſame ſpecific Religion) differ greatly in their Opinions of it.----*Laudatur ab his culpatur ab illis*.---Thoſe extol it to the Skies.---Theſe condemn it as the Spawn and Produce of Hell.----But as to my own particular Opinion of the Matter,——when I conſider the Practice of Inoculation,----and when I oppoſe the Benefits and Advantages which generally attend it, to the ſmall Riſk and Inconveniency of it,——it appears to me under ſeveral am-

ple

ple Attributes, or Characters;----and when I revolve in my Mind,---- and attentively survey---the Whole---the diffuse Sphere of Religion,---as well natural as revealed,——I can neither find in, nor deduce from the Whole any Thing that amounts to an Inhibition of this Practice.

As the first Law and express Voice of God (to us) was to increase and multiply,—so the first Law and express Dictate of Nature, is Self-Preservation.——Now by this Law, and Dictate of Nature, we are not to understand, barely and simply our Existence here.——But (subordinate to that) it also bids us take Care, and provide, to live sociably, comfortably, and happily.——To all which desirable Ends and Purposes, I assert, that the Practice of Inoculation, is a very great Accessory or Means.——This last Position is a self-evident Truth, and therefore stands in need of no Arguments or Reasonings to defend and support it.——In my Opinion of Things,—a Man void of Fear may be happy,—at least, 'tis a good Ingredient, and a very necessary one toward Happiness,——Tho' an acute Sense and Discernment of Things are also requisite.——Thus *Virgil* says,

Fælix Qui potuit Rerum dignoscere Causes
Atque Metue omnes; atque irresistabile Fatum
Subjecit Pedibus.——

But on the other Hand, a Person fetter'd with Fears and Terrours cannot possibly be happy or easy under them.

As to the abstract Idea, or Nature, of Inoculation,— I apprehend 'tis altogether as reasonable to suppose that the Almighty, All-gracious, and All-merciful Being did —— either actually and expresly inspire Mankind with it—or else supernaturally impress'd it on Mankind, for their Preservation, Comfort, and Happiness,——as that it occurr'd to us spontaneously,——or (in other Words) that it is a Child of mere Human Invention and Caprice;——so that, perhaps, the Thing called Inoculation may have a Right to boast a supernatural Descent or Degree, *i. e.* it may, perhaps, be a Thing of Divine Institution,——or at least may be the Result and Effect of a Divine Impulse,—— and not be a sordid Thing of mere Human Conceit and Contrivance.——But to support and admit the contrary of this, is it not manifest and notorious, that we bleed, we purge, and practise many other Means and Medicines in order to preserve Health, and prevent the Access of Diseases? The Practice of Inoculation was instituted, and is prosecuted to answer the same Ends and Purposes.—— —Plain Reason and common Policy instruct us, that it is better, and more eligible, to incur, or undergo, a slight Evil and Danger, which we might possibly avoid, than expose ourselves to the Risque of a much greater, which perhaps we cannot escape. And to this invariable and salutary Maxim it is that Inoculation (considered as a Human Invention) appeals for its Justification.

THE foregoing Objection is purely Theological; or rather Metaphysical:——But the following is strictly Physical; and therefore I may probably be the better qualified to dissect and display it in a proper Light. To that I now proceed—in which I will endeavour to be as brief and concise (taking Care at the same Time to be clear and explicite) as possible.——

AND

AND, *First*, That the Stamina, or Seeds of the Pox, a Scurvy, a Scropula, or of any other of the Distempers enumerated above, may be innate and inherent, or latent and concealed, in the Habit or Blood of the Person from whom the inoculating Matter is taken.—So far is very possible.

Secondly, THAT some small Portion or Part of the supposed latent Seeds, or Stamina, may be taken, together with the variolous Matter, and transplanted into the Habit of the Person inoculated—that also is somewhat probable——But what may we reasonably suppose to result from, or be the Consequence of all this? Why truly nothing at all.——This at least is my Sentiment upon the Matter. Nor is it possible, humanly speaking, that any Thing should result from it.

FOR, *Thirdly*, We must suppose the foreign Seeds, or Stamina, thus transplanted, are so very small, I mean in Quantity, as to be of no comparative Weight or Force—and consequently it is by far more reasonable to imagine that they will be vanquished, and as it were annihilated, by the Force of the Constitution, or the Animal Powers, into which they are received, than that, in their new Mansion, they should recover or acquire Force and Power enough to wage War upon it; and finally to reduce it under their Tyranny and Subjection.

Fourthly, and *lastly*, IT is very probable, and almost certain, that the whole Bulk of the supposed latent Seeds, which Bulk is infinitely small, is so wrought upon during the Progress of the Disease, by the variolous Fever, which both precede and ſometimes accompany it, either by dividing or comminuting their Molœcula or Parts; or elſe by digeſting and concocting them, as greatly to enervate and weaken their Force, if not entirely deſtroy their Eſſence.

But the Reaſonableneſs and Reſemblance of this Conjecture will obtain a yet greater Sanction, Authority and Force, if we only reflect on what is very obvious to daily Experience and Obſervation--- namely, that many Perſons who were, before they had the Small Pox, in the natural Way, valetudinary, weak, and ſickly—have nevertheleſs become healthy, robuſt, and ſtrong, upon their having paſs'd through that Diſeaſe.——And this, I think, proves plainly that the ſuppoſed ſick Perſons were (till they had had the Small Pox) incumbered and diſtreſſed—kept weak and ſickly—by Means of ſome inherent (though latent and inviſible) ill Habits, and that upon the Acceſs of the Small Pox—the ſuppoſed latent Seeds, or morbid Stamina, were intirely vanquiſhed, deſtroyed, and exterminated —— together with the variolous Fomes, or Principle—— But further — I muſt obſerve, that the ſuppoſed latent Seeds, or morbid Stamina (upon the Suppoſition of which this grand Objection is founded) are always ſubjected to two different Trials — or are twice put to the Torture.— And therefore if the firſt ſhould not perfectly meliorate and correct them — nor intirely deſtroy or ſubdue their noxious Qualities — yet their being ſoon after ſubjected a ſecond Time to the ſame Proceſs will, in Moral Certainty, compleatly effect it — For, *Firſt*, The variolous Matter (or Buds, as they are ſtiled) intended for the Purpoſe of Inoculation, is not taken out of the Puſtules till they are arrived at

a State

a State of Maturity— or nearly ſo. —And therefore any foreign (though latent) morbid Seeds or Stamina of other Diſeaſes, muſt neceſſarily be much weakned, and infeebled —if not intirely vanquiſhed and ſubdued. —And then the ſame foreign Seeds or Stamina of other Diſeaſes, are preſently deſtined to go through the whole Proceſs, and the ſame Torture again,— in the Conſtitution, or Habit of the Perſon, into which they have been thus tranſfuſed.——So that here I preſume they cannot fail to be utterly deprived, and to be even diveſted of Exiſtence—I mean as to any noxious morbid Quality——And thus I preſume (and I believe it will appear ſo to every candid, rational, unprejudiced Perſon) that this ridiculous Objection is intirely defeated.——In fine,—If I had ever ſo many Relations and Friends (of ſuch as never had the Small-Pox) whoſe Lives, Comfort and Happineſs, I was anxious and ſolicitous to preſerve, I would adviſe all, and each Individual of them, to be inoculated, for it is only undergoing a very light (though certain Inconvenience, and a mere Shadow of Danger, in order to elude a much greater (though uncertain one) of both Sorts.

The great Benefits and Advantages of Inoculation conſiſt chiefly in theſe two Articles.——1. In the previous Management and Preparation of the Perſon who is to be inoculated. And this with Regard to Diet, as well as Medicine. 2. In having the Matter for Inoculation taken from one who has a very mild, favourable Sort of Pox. And to theſe we may add, 3. That the beſt and propereſt Seaſon of the Year may be made Choice of, for undergoing of the Operation. And even this is no inconſiderable Article. In Conſequence of

theſe

prudent Cautions and Proceedings (and I hope no one would be ſo blind to his own Intereſt and Safety as to be inoculated, without being duly and judiciouſly prepar'd for it) every one, almoſt univerſally, who is inoculated, has a very mild and favourable Sort of Pox. In a Word, the abovementioned Benefits and Advantages that attend the Practice of Inoculation, when judiciouſly conducted, are obvious to, and avowed by, every candid, rational, and unprejudiced Perſon.

Now, to bring Inoculation in Contraſt with the natural or ſpontaneous Small Pox—The Difference will be not only very obvious, but very great alſo. For, *Firſt*, 'Tis very notorious, that every Perſon who takes the Small Pox in the natural Way is in Danger of his or her Life. *Secondly*, By the Inexorable Malice of this deadly Tyrant, Parents are often depriv'd of thoſe dear, invaluable Bleſſings, their Children;—And Children, *vice verſa*, of their dear, tender, indulgent Parents; Huſbands of their Wives, and Wives of their Huſbands.— And, *Thirdly*, of ſuch as fortunately go through it, and ſurvive it.——What Miſeries and Calamities are not many of them ſubjected to, even under the Progreſs of the Diſeaſe?——Beſides thoſe that ſometimes follow after,——how many fair blooming Faces, amongſt the tender, lovely Sex, have been deflower'd and cancell'd by it? How many Perſons have loſt their Eyes (ſome one, ſome both) by it? And of this I myſelf have known many melancholy Inſtances.———

Tho' I never (as above obſerv'd) concerned myſelf perſonally in conducting the Buſineſs of Inoculation,—as I never had the Small Pox, yet I am am very well instructed in, and acquainted with all the preparatory Methods at this Time in Practice.———And though the Preparatory Methods used, have (within the Space of ten or fifteen Years past) been very much improved,—and are at this present Time evidently good,—yet it is my Opinion, that I could superadd to them, and improve upon them a good deal.———

Be it not imagined, that I mention this with a View or Desire to be concern'd in the Practice of what I so earnestly recommend——(for I would much rather be excused from it); but I mention it in order to render the Practice of it yet more easy, safe, and salutary. And whosoever shall contribute, or whatsoever Advices may for the future contribute, to the Advancement and Improvement of the Methods at present known and practised,—will, I fancy, be thought to deserve well of the Publick.——But, for my own Part, I am soon going out of the Country—at least for a considerable Time;—and it is not certain that I shall return hither again. But, even, if my Views were so selfish and so sordid, as to hope and desire to reap Profit from and by the Practice of what I so strenuously recommend——I dare say I should be grosly disappointed——For I see clearly and plainly that the major Part of Mankind, in this Part of our Hemisphere, are so far prejudiced in Favour of certain Medical Idols (whose Sanctity and Excellencies are, perhaps, rather imagined or imputed than real and solid). as justly to incur the Censure of Infatuation—or Wrongheadedness. But to return to the Subject of Inoculation—this same Practice of Inoculation is not only a Benefit and a Blessing to Individuals, and to particular Communities and

and Societies— but 'tis likewise a Benefit to the State or Nation in general.—For, without all Peradventure, if this Practice was universally adopted, and prosecuted throughout the King's Dominions, many Thousands of his Majesty's Subjects would annually be preserved by it——And since Mr. *Paul* the Surgeon (who is a Person of considerable Fortune, as well as of distinguishing Ability and Eminence in his Profession) has as above observed, open'd the Scene, and commenced the Practice of it in these Parts——so I hope and expect that it will make a rapid Progress and Advance—— I have at this Time, and upon this Occasion, considered the Business of Inoculation with some Attention, and am really persuaded that I could (as above observ'd) superadd to, and improve upon, the preparatory Methods at present known and practised very considerably——However, for the present, I will say no more upon that Head—only offer a Suggestion (to Physicians and others who undertake the Business of Inoculation) whether the *Cortex* (given after proper Cooling and Cleansing, for a few Days before the Patients begin to sicken, and during the Progress of the Distemper) might not be of Use and Benefit.

Dr. WALL, a very judicious and accurate Physician at *Worcester*, has experienced it under some dangerous Circumstances of the natural and spontaneous Small Pox, with very great Success—as he intimates in a Piece he publish'd in the *Gentleman's Magazine* for *November* last. And as Dr. *Wall*'s Opinion upon the Matter quadrates exactly with my own Sentiments upon it— so I wrote a Piece, in order to the further Prosecution, Illustration, and Inforcement, of the same laudable and useful

Scheme,

Scheme, which is in the *Gentleman's Magazine* for laſt Month—which Piece is addreſs'd by way of Letter to Dr. *Wall*, and ſign'd *C. P.* But upon peruſing the ſaid *Magazine* the other Day—I find that the Compilers of the *Magazine* have curtail'd and abridg'd that Piece, ſo as to reduce it within leſs than half its Compaſs.—— I likewiſe find that Dr. *Cameron* (another very learned and judicious Phyſician at *Worceſter*) has publiſh'd a Piece upon much the ſame Subject in the *Gentleman's Magazine* for *January* laſt——but I did not meet with that till my Piece was gone to *London*, otherwiſe I had ſome proper Remarks and Obſervations to make upon it.——I am perſuaded that the learned and ingenious Dr. *Huxam* of *Plymouth* would be very well pleaſed with this Thought of giving the *Cortex*, upon inoculating the Small Pox.—And with all or either of theſe three ingenious Gentlemen (Dr. *Wall*, Dr. *Cameron*, and Dr. *Huxam*) I ſhould be very glad to confer upon this Subject; as well as upon ſome other Matters which my Studies within a few Days paſt have ſuggeſted to me.—— if I ſhould (after I have finiſh'd my Affairs at *London*) return back into this Country, and ſhould continue to enjoy the happy *Sine-Cure*, which I have been bleſs'd with for about ſix or ſeven Months (till within about three Weeks paſt, that it has indeed ſuffered ſome ſmall Interruption) I may in that Caſe very probably pay a Viſit to one or other of them.——I am not indeed acquainted with either of theſe Gentlemen,——nevertheleſs I very well know their Characters, and much eſteem their great Merits. ——Dr. *Wall* and Dr. *Cameron* are, I well know, very learned and ingenious Gentlemen.— And Dr. *Huxam* (as appears by the learned and elaborate Works which he has pub-

 liſhed)

lished) has deserved highly of the Medical Art and Faculty.——This Gentleman is a close and just Imitator of the great *Hippocrates*, and indeed seems to have transfused the whole Soul of that divine Antient into himself.——As I am very soon going to leave this Country—at least for a considerable Time—it is, I think, very proper and requisite that I make up Accounts with People before I depart.——And to that End and Purpose I can't omit to acquaint them, that a few Nights ago, I called and spent an Hour or two with a Family of my Acquaintance: The Chief of the Family (who is a very sensible Man, and my good Friend) seem'd to me to be sorry I was going to leave the Country, and supposing that the Cause of my leaving it was a Decay, or rather a total Desertion of my Practice. He told me, that he very well knew, and would clearly explain to me, the Causes of it.——And this he accordingly did in Manner following, *i. e.* My Friend reminded me, that at, or about, ten Months ago, I was consulted for a Woman (a very worthy and amiable Person she was) very far gone in a Waste or Consumption,—of which she soon after died——That a Person in the last Stage of a Consumption, should die, even under the Care and Advice of a Physician (supposing him to be the best and greatest in the World) that, you'll say, is no Wonder; and consequently, you'll say, I deservedly incurr'd no Censure and Reproach upon that Score.

Now, to speak my real Sentiments upon this Matter; or rather to say what I know for certain, This same good and lovely Woman died tabid, *i. e.* of a confirmed Tabes; which is a Distemper that generally proves fatal. And besides, it appear'd pear'd very plain to me, that her Blood and Juices were reduced to a very poor, ſpiritleſs, vapid State or Condition.—What then, in God's Name (People will naturally ſay) can be the Reaſon or Foundation for all the Cenſure, Calumny, and Slander which has been ſo induſtriouſly ſpread abroad? Seeing the Patient was ſo far gone, and reduced to ſo deplorable a State before I was called to her Why this is the very Caſe,—namely,—her tender, affectionate indulgent Mother (whom I look upon to be a very good and valuable Woman) was very inquiſitive and ſolicitous to know my Opinion and Thoughts as to the State of the Viſcera, and of the Lungs in particular.——In Anſwer to her importunate Queſtions and Enquiries (after I had examined what ſhe ſpit up) I gave it as my Opinion, that her Lungs were not ulcerated. Now, when ſuch appears to be the State of the Caſe, *viz.* that the Lungs are ulcerated, we then look upon our Patients to be one Remove (tho' perhaps but a ſmall one) from a State of Deſperation. At the ſame Time I neither did nor could, in my private Opinion, intirely diſculpate her Lungs, or ſuppoſe them quite undiſtemper'd: For 'tis well known to Phyſicians of good Judgment and Experience, that the Lungs (tho' quite free from Ulceration) may be affected and diſtempered various other Ways,—and ſuch as will with equal Certainty terminate in Death.

Upon the Death of this very excellent and amiable Creature, it was buz'd, or rather bellow'd abroad, as I am now inform'd, tho' I never heard a Syllable of it before, that I was moſt groſly miſtaken in her Diſtemper, for that I had declared her in a Way of Recovery, and as it were out of Danger,

ger, even the Day before ſhe died, and from theſe Premiſes it was inferr'd and concluded, that I muſt neceſſarily be very ignorant and quite deſtitute of ſound Judgment, and a good Diſcernment in Diſeaſes,—ſeeing that I had erred ſo very groſly in my Judgment upon this Caſe.

Now, in Anſwer to all this, I declare and aver, that the Whole, and every Part of the Accuſation, are abſolutely falſe in Fact; and conſequently that all the malicious Rumours and Reports which have been ſpread abroad are rank Calumny and Slander; —that they are equally black and baſe,—equally ſcandalous and villainous in their Nature; and I look upon all ſuch as have been concern'd in hatching, forging, ſpreading, and propagating theſe ſlanderous Reports — as infernal Imps; as mere Hell-hounds, *&c. &c. &c.*——But ſhould I deſcend from the metaphyſical Region, and give them ſome earthly Appellation—I am at a Loſs by what Name, Stile, or Title, to dignify and diſtinguiſh them—ſhall I pronounce them Wretches, Reptiles, or Harpies?

I FURTHER declare, and aver, that when I was firſt called to this amiable Creature (with whoſe Sweetneſs, and Lovelineſs I was quite charmed—and conſequently was very anxious to relieve, and recover her) I judg'd the Caſe to be extreamly dangerous; and to afford but ſmall Hopes of a Cure.——But I agree with *Celſus*—and will always follow his Maxim—in this—*viz.* Tho' a Diſtemper be ever ſo dangerous,—if not abſolutely deſperate——I will yet endeavour, and do my utmoſt for the Benefit of my Patient——even at the Riſque of my own Reputation.—And this is what a

Physician whose Views are sordid and selfish will scarcely do—lest the Issue of the Case should reflect Censure and blame upon him.

I FURTHER declare, That (whereas it is confidently reported that I gave Hopes of her Recovery even the Day before she died,) I did not see her, nor call upon her for several Days (I believe four or five) before she died.——How far her Mother (whom, as above observ'd, I look upon to be a good and valuable Woman) was concern'd in suggesting these Things—I don't know indeed,---but if she had any share in it---I can and do readily forgive her,---for I consider that she was, and necessarily must be, extremely afflicted and concern'd for the Loss of so excellent and amiable a Daughter. However the Access of this News to me, reminds me that her Mother (ever since her Daughter's Death) has very carefully shun'd the Sight of me, ---and has most scrupulously avoided me when ever she has seen me coming that way.

THIS, indeed, I often saw---and often observ'd ---but alas! I imputed it to quite another Cause. I imagin'd that this good Woman (my Patient's Mother) only regretted the Half Guiney she gave me when I was first called, (which was all I had of her; tho' I visited the Patient I believe half a Dozen Times) and that she thought it was all Money thrown away, as her Daughter was not recovered by it.

I WOU'D not have People infer, from what I have just now been saying, that I am so superabundantly modest in my Expectations and Demands. On the contrary, my Temper, is, perhaps,

haps, to be as ſaucy; and to put as high a Value upon my Services, as the proudeſt of the Faculty. But ſhou'd any one aſk me why I do not. I wou'd Anſwer as *Horace* did upon another Occaſion——*Cupidum, Pateroptime, vires deficiunt.* A Man muſt be poſſeſs'd of an Ample, or at leaſt an eaſy, Fortune to take ſuch a bold Step.——This however is a trite Politic which has been tried many a Time,---and with very happy Succeſs. ---For if one Doctor will inſiſt on Two Guineas for what another (of equal, perhaps ſuperior, Merit and Ability) will do for one.——The ignorant ill judging Part of Mankind will run with the greateſt Avidity after the former, becauſe they imagine his Advice muſt be twice as good as anothers.——The penetrating Eyes of the *French* would preſently ſee through and detect this Cheat. They would ſay,——*C'eſt pour s'encherir:* And in Truth I wonder the *Engliſh* don't ſee through it alſo. But God bleſs every Body—*i. e.* the Otherwiſe as well as the Wiſe.——But ſo much for a faſhionable Digreſſion—and I now gather up the Thread of my Narration. I muſt not forget to obſerve that the Minters and Propagators of the forementioned ſcandalous Reports, have acted with ſuch a Zeal and Indefatigableneſs as are ſcarce to be conceived or expreſs'd;——for in order to corroborate and validate their Slanders and Calumnies, upon this particular Affair, they have ſought after, and brought upon the Carpet other Things, as collateral Aids and Supports. Perhaps, indeed, they minted, and vented theſe others Slanders and Calumnies, not only as collateral Aids and Supports to the former, but alſo to revive and perpetuate them in People's Memories. —And if this was (as ſeems very probable) really the Caſe—then it muſt be confeſs'd they Acted

like

like very ſhrew'd (tho' puny) Politicians——but now to the Matter in Hand.

THOSE Hellhounds (my Perſecutors) have given out that my Conduct and Practice, in the Caſe of a Gentleman (whom I much Eſteem, Reſpect and Honour) was highly erroneous and blameable—or rather egregiouſly bad, abſurd and prepoſterous. ——That is to ſay,—in their Opinions of it;—and ſuch, doubtleſs, are the Marks and Characters they wou'd have repreſented it under——if they cou'd have fallen upon theſe Terms, or Expreſſions——however, they declared *(vivâ voce)* and and maintained *(totus viribus)* that I had certainly been the Death of that worthy Gentleman, if, by a lucky Incident, foreign Aid and Aſſiſtance had not ſeaſonably been called in, by whoſe Means (as they give out and maintain) the Gentleman was happily reſcued from the imminent Perils and Dangers I had brought him into.—And whereas it is (or at leaſt was at that Time) notorious that my Brethren and I differ'd very widely in our Opinions concerning the Nature of the Diſtemper, and the Methods proper to be uſed,—I here aſſert, and claim to myſelf, the whole and ſole Merit of that Cure—and this I will maintain againſt all Oppoſers whatever. And if I was to attempt a Recognition and Recital of the whole Caſe,—from the Beginning to the End,—with my Sentiments upon it, and Proceedings in it,—and offer them to the Publick,—I believe they would do me both Credit and Honour in the Opinions and Judgments of the more diſcerning and unprejudiced Part of the Faculty—I ſo fully and clearly ſaw the erroneous Opinions of my Colleagues concerning this Caſe, that I thought it incumbent on me (for my own Credit and Ho-

nour

nour) to declare my Diſſention from them.—And I now recollect, that once upon that Occaſion, a very agreeable worthy young Lady (out of pure Friendſhip and Kindneſs to me) adviſed me by all Means rather to conceal than confeſs to the World my diſagreeing with my Colleagues upon this Caſe. As ſhe imagined the Knowledge of it might diſcredit me in the Eſtimation and Opinion of the World.—But (ſo obſtinate and opiniated was I, or ſo it might be thought I was) that I diſdained and deſpiſed any ſuch baſe Compliances.

INDEED this Affair deſerves to be more fully diſſected and diſplayed— and this I could and would do pretty effectually,—if I thought it would not be diſagreeable to the very worthy Gentleman who was the Subject of it.—I remember it was with much ado I could reſtrain myſelf from writing and publiſhing the whole Proceedings in the Caſe as ſoon as it was ended.—And the very ſame Reaſons which would alone prevent me now, did ſo at that Time.—But was I to exhibit at large a true and faithful Narrative of the whole Proceedings and Machinary—*i. e.* to repreſent all the Stratagems, Intrigues and Devices of my Confederates in the Caſe, they would amount at leaſt to a good Farce, and by the Help of a little Elbow-greaſe, would make a good Comedy.—Judge only, *Firſt*, How I muſt be ſurprized to ſee a young Gentleman, though in Truth a very ſenſible one, ſent from afar off to aſſiſt me in a Conſultation. And then, *Secondly*, To ſee all the Confidence and Truſt transferred from me to him,—whereas it was moſt manifeſt, that this Gentleman was really, with reſpect to Years and Experience, a mere Suckling, compar'd to myſelf.—But then, whereas

whereas it was plain that this Gentleman was but of late Years initiated in the τα̉ἱπορʼγητα, the ſacred Myſteries, and the Practice of Medicine——and in order to ſupport and confirm to him the Prehemi-nence——another Gentleman (one of a more ma-ture Age) was joined with him——ſo that under this happy Aſſociation and Combination they could and did carry all before them——I ſaw immediate-ly and very plainly, that I had nothing more to do than to be a Spectator: To ſignify my Acquieſ-cence by my Silence——and to ſpecify my Aſſent by my Signature----and this I did, indeed, ſeeing that nothing I could propoſe was admitted, and that nothing which they advanced could be deſtructive or pernicious. In reality it was very plain to me, that our worthy Patient was quite out of Danger before any of theſe Gentlemen were called in to my Aſſiſtance, and would have been much ſooner reſtored to perfect Health, if they had never come to my Help.

THIS Affair was ſpread and blazed about the Country for many Miles around,—and as I very well remember, much to my Prejudice and Detri-ment,—I was told, with a Note of Admiration and Aſtoniſhment, by ſeveral Gentlewomen, my good and worthy Friends, many Miles hence, that Doctor ſuch a one had taken the Precedence of me in Conſultation, by ſigning firſt.

IN good Truth, when the ſaid Gentleman and myſelf were firſt concern'd together, which was in another and preceding Caſe, I did pay him the Complement of Precedence——little thinking he would accept it——and not renumerate any Po-liteneſs, by a Tender of the ſame Civility—but ſo it happened, that he accepted of it as his undoubted Right then—and has ever ſince aſſumed it. But I have been long ſince reſolv'd, if ever we meet in Conſultation again, to enquire into his Pretenſions to this Right of Precedence.— Be it underſtood, however, that the Right of Precedence, with us, does not depend upon Superiority of Merit, or Superiority of Years,—but upon a prior Date of our Commiſſion.——I muſt not omit to mention, that the youngeſt of my Colleagues (who, though an Alien, was the Phyſician Reſident) on the Morning before he departed, gave a long Preſcription into my Hands, which he had doubtleſs drawn up proviſionally for that Purpoſe, and graciouſly deſign'd as a Rule for me to walk by.

When I return'd home in the Evening, I look'd it over, but found little or nothing in it that I could approve—ſome Things indeed that I much diſapprov'd.—— Upon this I put Pen to Paper, and drew out a Sketch of my own Thoughts upon the Matter.——And this (with his own) I gave into the Gentleman's Hands, for his Peruſal, the next Morning — A little before he departed, he look'd it over with a ſlight Air,——then return'd it to me, ----and ſoon after ſet out for his Abode——But, to my very great Surprize, on the Evening of this ſame Day came the other Phyſician to ſee our Patient. Well then (ſaid I to myſelf) 'tis very plain I cannot be truſted one Day; no, not one Hour. I was indeed cited *(pro formâ)* at this, and other ſubſequent Times, to come in Conſultation with this Colleague——But as I ſaw plainly that our Patient had nothing to do but to grow gradually in Health and Strength, ſo I gave very little Attention either to or at our Meetings. I don't at all queſtion

but

but that the young Gentleman, when he return'd home, and was ask'd by the Friends of our Patient, how he left him? answered, that he left him in a very good Way,—and that he did not doubt but he would do very well——if no unlucky fatal Mistake were futurely by me committed. But shall I stop here? No! I cannot! I must go on further. —This infernal Crew, my Slanderers, have attempted to draw fresh Recruits and Succours (in order to give a keener Edge, as well as greater Force and Effect to their villainous Calumnies) from my Conduct in the Illness of a young Lady, whose Death I cannot think of without the extremest Regret and Concern (as she was truly a very lovely engaging Person) upon this melancholy Occasion, they have minted and vented a thousand Calumnies and Slanders—and such as I can't hear or think of without being as much astonished at the Fruitfulness of their Invention, as at their Villainy and Impudence.

In Answer to these Censures and Slanders, my Friend (who is a sensible worthy Man) said; that to his certain Knowledge both the Families had declar'd themselves perfectly well satisfied as to my Conduct in both Cases—— and that they believed I had done all that was possible for a good Physician to do. To this they (my Persecutors) replied,— They (meaning the Families) might perhaps say so—but what (themselves) said was the Truth.--- Thus they, in Fact, charge these worthy Families with Prevarication and Falshood.——And suppose that the Language of their Tongues, and the Thoughts of their Hearts, differ as widely as Black from White——by this they insinuate, that though both the Families are fully persuaded and convinced

 of

of my Errors and Miſtakes,—yet out of a humane compaſſionate Diſpoſition, they had rather draw a Veil over, and conceal them, than ruin my Character by expoſing them.——But further, theſe Wretches have given out that a certain Perſon (a very near Ally to the Family) damn'd me, and that he otherways inſulted and abuſed me in a very groſs and outrageous Manner —— And that I, being conſcious and convinced of my Errors and Miſtakes, took it very calmly and contentedly, which, however, is ſomewhat alien from my natural Temper.

As concerning this laſt Article,—this, indeed, does ſeem to have ſome Shadow of Foundation; for, though the whole, and every Part of this Aſſertion is abſolutely falſe in Fact,—yet I muſt acknowledge it (and ſorry I am that I am oblig'd to mention it, but I dare not omit it, becauſe ſhould I deny any one Article which they can make appear to have ſome Shadow of Foundation——they would not fail to exult and triumph upon it, and would palm all the reſt of their deviliſh Lies upon the World for Truths. That Gentleman, who is a very worthy, ſenſible, and well-bred Man, did once ſo far forget himſelf, or, to uſe the Expreſſion of *Shakeſpear*, was ſo far wide of his own Reſpect, as to expreſs himſelf ſomewhat indecently, which, however, though I can't well forget it, I readily forgive.

Now leſt theſe Folks, my Perſecutors, ſhould be under any Fears or Apprehenſions that their baſe, villainous Slanders have not had the deſired Effect, I do hereby, and by theſe Preſents, certify, and declare, that their zealous and impious En-

deavours

deavours to ruin my Reputation have met with all the Succeſs they could wiſh or deſire; for during the Space of ſix or ſeven Months paſt, till very lately, my Practice has greatly decay'd,--- or rather totally deſerted me.——I hope my Perſecutors will think themſelves obliged to me for this Information—and that they'll have as much Pleaſure in the Reading, as I have in the Relating it.

My good Friend (who reveal'd theſe Secrets to me) declar'd that he believ'd that I had loſt at leaſt an hundred Guineas, nay, much more, within leſs than a Year paſt, in Conſequence of theſe ſlanderous Reports. Indeed he mention'd ſeveral particular Perſons——who wou'd have ſent for me, if they had not been terrified and hinder'd by the baſe and villainous Stories, that were then current of me.—But ſo it did (as moſt probably it wou'd) fall out——when my Merits and Accompliſhments were ſuperceded and ſet aſide.— They then ſent, the Lord knows where, for the Lord knows who, in Quality of a Phyſician.---- Perhaps, indeed, theſe Calumnies and Slanders were coined and utter'd againſt me with no other View and Deſign, than to ſtrip me of every Merit, and every Accompliſhment——and then to lay what they had robb'd and deſpoil'd me of, upon the Back of another—who perhaps may ſtand in need of them.

We very well know, that there is a certain medical High Prieſt, who (with the more illiterate and undiſcerning Part of Mankind) is highly celebrated and reverr'd——to whoſe loaden Altars the Generality of old Women (of both Sexes) pay the profoundeſt Adoration, and are inceſſantly offering

fering Incenſe.——And yet (notwithſtanding theſe prepoſterous Prejudices, of an ill judging wrong-headed People) I had within leſs than a Year ago, ſo well diſtinguiſhed myſelf, by ſeveral very happy and great Cures, in very arduous and difficult Caſes.—That ſome of my Friends complimented me upon the Proſpect and ſure Preſages of an approaching Increaſe of Fame and Renown.——Theſe Perſons (my Friends) argu'd in my Favour, that I ſhou'd, and neceſſarily muſt, very ſoon blaze out in full Luſtre, and come into great Fame and Practice.——But how much (alas) are Times chang'd——with us? And Opinions and Expectations——with them.——And hence it ſhould ſeem to be with Phyſicians as (according to the Poet's Expreſſion) it is with the Fair Sex, —*i. e.* one falſe Step (whether real or only imputed) intirely damn's our Fame.———Now it having been plainly and clearly made appear to me, that theſe baſe, villainous Slanders, and Calumnies have caus'd me the Loſs of ſome certain Patients.—-I can't help ſuſpecting that ſome other Defections and Deſertions have ſprung from the ſame Source.

Now, by Means of the new Lights, which reſult to me from theſe Informations, I can form probable Conjectures concerning certain Phænomena; which otherwiſe I ſhou'd ſcarce be able to account for and explain,—and of theſe I cannot omit (how diſagreeable ſoever the mentioning them may be to me) to relate the moſt remarkable and ſtriking.—And (*Firſt*,) There is a very worthy and hopeful young Perſon, (one of a very conſiderable Family in this Place,——of a Family whom I was always in very good Friendſhip with,

----and

—and had I think a very good Right to be held in Preference by them to any other Physician hereabouts) who was much indisposed about seven or eight Months ago.---Now it came to pass, (for so the Fates wou'd have it) that the good People (his Relations and Friends) quite forgetting me, or overlooking me, sent out, *quaque versum*, to remote Places in quest of Physicians. *First*, (according to Custom) they sent for one; who is a Gentleman of good Sense, and a good Physician doubtless.——But alas! after they had used him some Time, and were grown weary of him) for so the Fates would have it) they left him, and sent the Lord knows where for another.----In, and with this their new Choice, they seem'd to acquiesce, and to rest perfectly satisfied,——as if this was the—*Ne plus ultra*—the last Resort. If this Man cou'd not cure him,—GOD's Will be done. And yet I very well remember, that, in those Days, some very wise Folks were of Opinion that they expos'd their Judgment to just Censure, by the Change and new Choice they had made; and intimated that they had honoured the old Proverb (*out of the Frying-Pan into the Fire*) with a plenary Accomplishment by it.—And besides, this same Freak or Frolick, of sending out to remote Places, for medical Assistance,—was not only more expensive to them, but more inconvenient also, on many Accounts. However, under the Auspices of this new Doctor, (who plyed the Patient very assiduously) the Patient languished a good while,—'till at length his Distemper was rather worn out by Time, (as some Folks imagine) than cured by Medicines.—But supposing that they had taken a Pique at, or been dissatisfied with, this last Doctor,—and that the

the Diſtemper had remain'd unconquer'd,—I dare ſay, they wou'd have ſent out to the remoteſt Corners of the Earth (Eaſt, Weſt, North and South) in queſt of Phyſicians,—rather than have conſulted me,—ſo that I muſt neceſſarily judge, and conclude, that I have been repreſented to them as a very dangerous Perſon.

I HAVE always look'd upon this as the moſt fatal Stroke to my Character and Eſtabliſhment here: For this Event muſt neceſſarily ſet all the People at a Gaze! It muſt make them ſtare and wonder! What in GOD's Name (People wou'd ſay) has Dr. *Perry* done——to incur ſuch a palpable Slight, and ſo groſs an Affront? And this from a Family in the Neighbourhood, with whom he was always well acquainted, and in good Friendſhip.

THERE is yet another Affair (that happen'd lately in a neighbouring Town) which appears very myſterious to me, and which I can't otherwiſe account for than by ſuppoſing it to ſpring from the ſame poiſonous Source.——There was a Gentlewoman (of a Family I was well enough known to) who was ſeiz'd with a Fever of which ſhe afterwards died.——Now, whereas I had very well diſtinguiſhed and ſignalized myſelf in and about that Town, by many happy and great Cures——ſo I might reaſonably imagine, and expect, that I ſhould be had in Preference there, to any other Phyſician——more eſpecially by all ſuch as I was either acquainted with or known to.——And beſides——this Gentlewoman had a Siſter with her (a Gentlewoman whom I had obliged, but the laſt Year, in a very eſſential

Point

Point, by remitting, or giving up, a Claim of at least five Guineas: - And I vow I wou'd not undergo the same Fatigue and Anxiety again for that Recompence) all the Time of her Illness,— and from whom I might reasonably expect that she wou'd (either out of her Opinion of my superior Skill, or out of Gratitude to my Generosity) have advised and recommended me to her Sister.—— But notwithstanding all these my Pretensions (whether real and substantial or only by me vainly imagined) to a Right of Preference,— they sent further off for another Physician—by and under whose happy Auspices, the Patient was, in God's good Time, safely consign'd to the peaceful Mansions of the Grave.——Be it not imagined, that I mean by what I have said, to undervalue or depreciate the Merits of the Person who was concern'd in the Case,——far otherwise,—for I profess to have a very good Opinion of him,—and a very good Esteem for him;——but as in the military Sphere the veteran Troops have always the Preference to those of a later Establishment, who are less experienced in the Art of War;-—— so in the Sphere of Physick, the oldest Officer should, I think, have the same.

A few Days ago a certain Person very officiously told me, that Miss such a one was in a very weak declining Way, &c. This Intelligence instantly called to my Remembrance, that betwixt two and three Years ago, I attended this same Person in a dangerous nervous Fever,—from which I happily recovered her.——I remember likewise, that being ask'd by the Parents (after my Patient was recovered) what Recompence I required or expected,—I referr'd it (as I wou'd gladly do in all Cases) to themselves to give what they pleased. ——However, they insisted that I shou'd say what wou'd content me. And seeing that I was indispensably oblig'd to be my own Carver, I resolved not to err, unless it was on the Right Side. Therefore I was so extreamly modest as to say one Guinea, accordingly one Guinea I had.——Tho' two or three wou'd have been nearer the Mark of my just Deserts.-——And, indeed, 'tis generally (tho' not always) my Way, when I am oblig'd to carve for myself, to leave room to superadd considerably,—but notwithstanding I was so successful, and withall so very moderate and disinterested in my Demand,—yet this same Person (in a subsequent Illness) quite overlook'd me; and has quite forgot the Justice and Gratitude she owed to my past Services. And, in fine, has been hawking about, the Lord knows where, for Advice.—— However, as this Act was prior in Date to the Invention and Dispertion of the fore mentioned Slanand Calumnies,—so I look upon the Defection, and Apostacy of this Person and her Adherents to be the pure Effect of a gross heavy Understanding;—and, perhaps, it might appear (upon a nice Scrutiny) that the Fauners and Worshipers of a certain Idol are, generally speaking, Persons of that Sort of Temperament.——In good Truth, the old Axiom (*Similia Similibus gaudent*) will most commonly claim the Sanction of its Accomplishment.——And very right it is that it shou'd be so,—for if old Axioms, and old Maxims, as well as old Phrophecies and Proverbs, were not to be frequently accomplished and fulfilled,—they wou'd very soon lose their Force and Credit,--- and be no more,----what they were.

I RE-

I REMEMBER, that in the first Days (not of my Reign but) of my Estabishment here, I perform'd several very great Cures in Cases of the Throncc kind ——All of them--- *Pro Deo*---and such as would have eternized any one Physician of an hundred.——And yet those signal Instances of my Success——those strong Indications of a superior Skill---were of no manner of Effect in the Extention of my Fame and Practice.

I HAVE (as may be made appear) perform'd many great Cures since I have been in this Country.——And of such the most remarkable, which at present occur to my Memory are *First*, that I perform'd upon *John Tyler* of *Beach Appearame*. *Secondly*, That upon *Sarah Grindall* of *Frampton-Green*. The *Third* was on honest *George Harmer* of *Ranwick*. And the *Fourth Richard White* of *Westripp*.——The first-mentioned (*John Tyler*,) had been grievously afflicted with a Bloody Flux, (attended with most excruciating Pains) for eight or nine Weeks——which had reduc'd him both in Body and Purse to the Brink of Destruction.

I WELL remember that *John Tyler* sent a Man of his Acquaintance, with a State of his Case in Writing, on Sunday in the Afternoon; and had addressed himself to my Predecessor;--but the Messenger, being come to the Top of the Town, met a Man of his Acquaintance, who ask'd him, What Business brought him to Town?—the Messenger told him, that he was come to request Doctor such a one's Advice for his Friend *John Tyler*, who was in a very weak deplorable Condition.——The Man reply'd, The Doctor has been dead and buried several Weeks.—What, alas! shall I do then for my poor sick Friend? answer'd the Messenger— The Person reply'd to him, that his Purpose nevertheless, might be at least as well serv'd, if not better; intimating, that tho' the other Doctor was dead, a much greater was come in his Place. ——One, said he, who is no less charitable and beneficient to the Poor and Needy,---than successful in every Thing he undertakes --Upon this Encouragement the Man came down to me; and shew'd me the State of the Case in Writing,—— which, indeed, was conceiv'd and express'd in very aukward uncouth Terms.

AFTER I had perus'd the Scripture, I told the Man, that as the Case seem'd to be very intricate and very dangerous, so I must necessarily see the sick Person, in order to do him effectual Service. That, Sir, reply'd the Man, is what we can neither expect nor desire: For, added he, the poor Man is very much reduced by his long Illness, and is quite unable to make you any Recompence —— That, said I, shall not break Squares —— I must, and will, see the poor Man, and will do it with as much Promptitude and Pleasure, as if he was the richest Person in the Country.—— Accordingly I went the next Morning; and after I had fully examined into the Case, and duly considered every Symptom and Circumstance of it, I then prescribed for him. Well! This very Prescription alone (which indeed was somewhat copious,—as it contained two distinct Processes of Medicine) perfectly cured and restor'd the Man to Health.--And I really look upon this to be as great a Cure as has been perform'd at any Time or Place. This Case I must confess was not strictly Speaking of the Chronic Kind, unless it may be stiled such on Account of its long

Con-

Continuance ;—but I assert that Chronic Cures are the best and surest Test of a Physician's Judgment and Skill—— for acute Diseases may terminate either in Death, or a perfect Recovery—without the Physician's being to blame in the former——or intitled to Praise in the latter——because in these Cases the best judg'd and best concerted Methods may be defeated by the Disease. As on the contrary, a happy and salutary Crisis shall sometimes be brought about under the most injudicious Treatment.

THE second Case I shall mention, is of one *Sarah Grindall* of *Frampton*. This poor Creature (who was then eleven Years of Age) was quite over-run with a scrophulous Disorder — the most inveterate and virulent I ever saw —— and such as would, I believe, (let Mr. *Chart* or who will, think otherwise) make a Mock at the Royal Touch— where, or in whomsoever this fancied Virtue might be reposed.—— In fine, this poor Girl was render'd a perfect Cripple—— she was brought by her Father in his Arms (being quite incapable of walking) to Mr. *Cambridge*'s House; at whose particular Instance and Request I examined the Case, and prescribed for her.——I very well remember that Mr. *Cambridge* told me, I might expect some Recompence for my Cure and Advice——but as the Case appeared to me almost desperate— so I absolutely disclaimed any Recompence, but promised to do her all the Service in my Power —*Pro Deo.*— I accordingly undertook her, and prescribed for her from Time to Time, and at length I recover'd her—— even beyond the most sanguine of my Hopes and Expectations.——I remember I called to see this Girl about a Year after, when

when ſhe was very well.——What may have befallen her ſince I don't know indeed.

Now I really imagined (ſo groſſy was I miſtaken in my Computation) that this ſignal Inſtance of my Succeſs——this ſo eminent and evident a Specification, or rather a Proof of a ſuperior Judgment and Skill—would have impreſs'd Mr. *Cambridge* with very favourable and advantageous Ideas of me, and more eſpecially as the Cure was performed upon ſo arduous and intricate a Caſe——upon a Diſeaſe which claims the firſt Place amongſt thoſe which are commonly ſtiled the *Opprobria atque flagella Medicorum*——But, alas! in this alſo it appears, I was groſſy miſtaken in my Computation:—For though I might very reaſonably flatter myſelf with the vain Conceit, that my great Succeſs, and my very generous and diſintereſted Behaviour in this Caſe, would entitle me to the Favour of that Gentleman, and would decree me the Preference in his Opinion to all other Phyſicians hereabout,—yet I never, to my Knowledge, received one ſpecific Mark of his Favour and Friendſhip.——Nor, indeed, thoſe Inſtances and Marks of Regard which (if I don't over-rate my Pretenſions) I am juſtly entitled to. I remember indeed, that I was ſent for to one *James Shaw*, a principal Workman to Mr. *Cambridge*——at a Time when Mr. *Cambridge* was from home.——In Event, this poor Man (for ſo the Fates would have it) died.——But I humbly conceive that was not through any Miſtake or Defect of mine.—— This was, as I well remember, a pulmonary Diſeaſe, and I had given the poor Man great Relief——but a ſudden and violent Irruption of freſh Matter upon his Lungs carried him off at once.——The like happened

to

to one *Edward Hyatt* but a few Months before—whom I had rescued and recovered from a similar Disorder to a Miracle.—— I well remember that I was very sparing of my Visits to *James Shaw*—that I might not incur too great Expence, as that must fall somewhere. But, Mr. *King*, Mr. *Cambridge*'s Steward, observing this, sent me a very pressing Letter, desiring I would not fail to give due Attendance; for that the Man was much valued by his Master— and I should be well recompensed for my Care and Trouble.——But even in this likewise I was much deceived in my Computation, and disappointed in my Expectations; for I was put off with one Guinea only, where I had very just Pretensions to Three.

BEFORE I quit the Region of *Frampton*, I must not omit to mention the Case of one Mr. *Bernard* of that Place, who came hither to consult me about the Month of *March*, either two or three Years ago—— upon the Recommendation of my very worthy and esteem'd Friend, *Samuel Hawker*, Esq;——This Man was greatly oppress'd with an Asthma, and deeply immersed in a Dropsy: He had been under the Care of another Physician for a Year before, but had reaped little or no Benefit. When he came first to consult me, his Apothecary, who came with him, brought several of the other Physicians Prescriptions——which seem'd, in my Opinion, to be not only inadequate to the Demands of the Case, but very ill-judg'd likewise. I asked the Patient how such, and such, and such particular Things agreed with him. He reply'd, that they disagreed with him very much—— that they did him no Manner of good——but, on the contrary, produced some bad Effects—— and such as I had an-

anticipately ſuppoſed. —— In fine, I preſcrib'd for him three Times, each at a Week's Diſtance from the other. The firſt Preſcription did him conſiderable Service. And the Second, tho' he uſed but one Half of the Medicines preſcrib'd, much more. And tho' he came a third Time to conſult me, and had a third Preſcription of me,—yet he was ſo much reliev'd and recover'd by the Firſt, and half the Second——that he ſet aſide half the Medicines of the Second---and never had the Third prepar'd. However, this Man did afterwards fall into ſome other Diſorder—— and notwithſtanding the eminent Service I had done him, was ſo far infatuated or bewitch'd as to ſend for his *quondam* Doctor,—— who ſoon put an End to his Sufferings and his Life together.

THE *Third* Caſe I have to mention is that of honeſt *George Harmer* of *Ranwick*, whom I reſcued and perfectly recover'd from a very intricate complicated, and terrible Diſtemper, of which however, I cannot now recollect all the Circumſtances.

THE *Fourth* remarkable Caſe, and Cure, which I ſhall mention, is of *Richard White* of *Weſtripp* ——whom I cur'd (by internal Means only) of an inveterate and virulent Cancer, that had almoſt demoliſh'd the Gnomon of his Face: Or (to ſpeak more intelligibly) that graceful Fabrick his Noſe, was almoſt eat away by it. Now one would really imagine that theſe four Cures (to go no further) might ſufficiently ſpecify of me, and teſtify for me,——and may, at leaſt, ſuppoſe of me, and for me, that I am equal, in Judgment and Skill, to the reſt of my Brethren.

MANY

MANY other Persons and Things (similar to what I have related) intrude themselves upon my Mind at this Crisis---and upon this Occasion,—— and they do somewhat impetuously, demand to be represented. But shou'd I undertake to recite them all; with the necessary and proper Remarks upon them—they would swell this Piece (which I design'd should be very short) to a Volume: And for that Reason I would willingly pass them all over in Silence.——However, my great Regard for Brevity must not hinder me from mentioning, that, even in this Country, I have performed surprising Cures in consumptive Cases.—Some of these I have perfectly recovered who had been look'd upon as incurable—and to several others, in whom there was an indelible tho' perhaps invisible Stain—such as it was not in the Power of the Medical Art or Medicine to wipe out, I have given very great and speedy Relief.——Now, I presume, every reasonable considerate Person will allow, that the Physician who gives the greatest and speediest Relief——even in such of those Cases as are not in their Nature cureable——would give a Patient the best Chance for his Recovery, where the Distemper will admit of it.——And here I shall take Leave to recite some Cases which I think are signal and flagrant Proofs of what I have been saying upon this Head. And,

First, ABOUT the Month of *February* was four Years, I was called to a young Man (about seventeen or eighteen Years old, as I guess) who had been for a long Time in a consumptive Way.—— I well remember that I visited and treated him, as well out of Regard to my own Reputation as for his Benefit, with great Care and Diligence, as it was in the first Days of my Establishment here.——

If I remember right, I visited him daily for about seven Weeks, and at length perfectly recover'd him. However, I remember very well, and to my Cost—that the Lad's Father asked me, after his Son was recover'd) what Recompence I requir'd?—and I told him, Half a Dozen Guineas.—Upon this the Wretch (his Father) ran babbling about the Country, telling every one he met, that I had made him pay me Six Guineas (though I never saw one Penny of his Money, or ever shall) for attending his Son a few Days only.——And thus this Wretch, by spreading such Lies about the Country, has been, as I am well inform'd, a great Detriment to me.

THE second Case of this Sort which I shall mention, was of a young Girl at *Stonehouse*, whom, (though in the last Stage of a Phthisis) I recover'd to a Miracle. However, she afterwards relapsed and died.

THE third Case is of one *Driver* of *Rodborow* Parish, for whom my Advice was desired in *October* last was two Years. I went on a *Sunday* Evening, as usual with me, to drink Tea with a Family of my Acquaintance—when the Gentlewoman of the House told me she had a Favour to request of me.——I reply'd, that she might command me in any Thing——and desired to hear what it was she had to request of me.——This worthy Gentlewoman (having prefaced her Request with some Apologies—and given me to understand that I should be recompenced) desired the Favour of me to look upon and give my Advice to a young Man who was in a consumptive Way.—I reply'd, that I would do the young Man all the

Service

Service in my Power, out of Respect and Regard to her Intercession and Recommendation, without Fee or Reward. Accordingly the young Man, who was provisionally order'd to be there for that Purpose, was brought in —I found him, indeed, upon Examination, pretty deeply immersed in a Consumption.——However, I thought, upon the whole, that the Case might admit of a Cure,—— seeing it did not appear to me that his Lungs were ulcerated.—— Having duly consider'd the Case, and consider'd of what was proper to be done in it, I prescrib'd for him.——This first Prescription, which directed a Process that was to last about a Fortnight, did him a great deal of Service.—— On that Day fortnight (going again to drink Tea with the same Family) the young Man was order'd there again to have my further Advice.——I then prescribed for him a second Time,—and this my second Prescription perfectly recover'd him; and it is my real Opinion, is as happy and speedy a Cure as ever was perform'd in the like Case. However, this same young Fellow, in the ensuing *Christmas* Holidays, which was about two Months after his Recovery, caught a violent Cold by sleeping on the Grass, after he had been carouzing with good Ale. And this falling upon his Lungs, occasioned a Relapse.—— Well, what was to be done now?—— Why, the Gentlewoman who had engaged my Advice for him before, well knowing that he had neither the Gratitude nor the good Manners to make me even the Offer of an Acknowledgment for my past Services, would not encourage nor countenance him in troubling me any more.

Now, it luckily came to pass, that a Gentleman in the Neighbourhood being indisposed, sent for a certain medical Apoſtle from afar off.—The young Fellow's Relations and Friends having Intelligence of this—they adviſed him by all Means to watch the Doctor's Coming,—and then to repair to the Gentleman's Houſe, to aſk the Doctor's Advice,-- which they did not at all queſtion but he might have—*gratis.*——Well, the young Man did ſo, and the Doctor preſcrib'd for him—*gratis*——as it was imagined. —— The ſame Doctor being called thither again ſome Time after,—— the young Man went thither to give him the Meeting, and got a ſecond Preſcription of him —And as he imagined the firſt was to coſt him nothing— ſo he thought he ſhould have the ſecond upon the ſame Terms.— But as the young Fellow was bruſhing off,— the Doctor (who is a wiſe Man, and who knows that, according to the Poet,

Of Sterling true One Thouſand Pounds ſupplies
The Want of Twenty Thouſand Qualities—)

ſaid to him—Stay young Man—you muſt give me before you go, two Half-Guineas for theſe two Naughts— alias Notes —only the Word was expreſs'd with a broad Accent, that it might make a deeper and ſtronger Impreſſion—I ſuppoſe. —The young Fellow was quite thunder-ſtruck at this Demand—and would gladly have been excuſed from complying with it.— However, the Doctor told him, he muſt and would have two Half-Guineas for theſe two Naughts.——But for the future he would give him this Advice *gratis* as often as he came to aſk it. —— Well, the poor young Man was forced to lug out —— thoſe precious Drops of his Heart's Blood——the two Half-Guineas.— But, alas! he did not live to trouble the

Doctor

Doctor any more. The second Prescription did his Business—it gave him the *Coup de Grace.* This put him out of all Manner of Pain, and committed him safely to the gloomy Regions of the Dead.

At or about this same Time, *William Maycott* (then in the Service of my good Friend *Thomas Daunt*, Esq;) came to ask my Advice for a Disorder that had violently seized his Lungs——insomuch that it was fear'd he was in a Consumption.—I only wrote once for him (and would take nothing, out of Respect to the Family he lived in, —tho' the honest Man offered me a Fee) and that Prescription perfectly cured him.

The last Case of this Kind which I shall mention, is, of honest Mr. *Pierce* of *Stinchcombe*.—— This worthy Man (for such he really was) had been ill, and under the Care of the great Metropolitan for the Space of about four Months before I was called to him; and he had, as it seem'd, reap'd no sort of Benefit.——There were no less than four very formidable Powers (a quadruple and terrible Alliance) that waged War upon him together—— namely, the Gout, Asthma, Dropsy, and Consumption.—— However, though it must be owned, that such a Combination and Confederacy was really very dreadful——yet I did, in four or five Times that I visited him, give him very surprising Relief in every Symptom and Circumstance of his Disorder.——I well remember that the last Time I visited this Person, I had the Pleasure to meet with my worthy Friend *William Townsend*, Esq; there,—upon whose Recommendation I was first concern'd for him ——I then found my Patient sitting by the Fire-side, and he both look'd

and

and talk'd very cheafully.—He told me, he had a tolerable good Appetite, and Relish to his Food; and, that he hoped by the Time we came that Way again, that he should be able to play a Game at Cards with us — at Whist — a Game he dearly loved:— But, after all—this very honest Man did, within some Time after, drop off at once, and died.

THERE is one Case more occurs to my Memory, which I shall take Leave to mention.——It is of a young Woman, an upper Servant in a House not far distant, to whom I was called soon after I came into these Parts. This young Woman's Disorder (which I think chiefly affected her Mouth) was very intricate, vexatious and inveterate. I well remember that I attended this Person several Days (about five or six, I believe) and in that Time I perfectly recover'd her,—at least for that Time,—Though I don't know what might happen to her after.—I remember likewise, that this Person told me (whilst I visited her) she had been under the Advice of another Physician for a considerable Time together; but had reap'd no Benefit from his Prescriptions. Now, probably the Physician, who preceeded me in this Case, might be recompenced for his intended Services;—but I had nothing for my real and effectual ones.——I must own, however, that the young Woman did come to me, several Weeks after she was cured, to make an Acknowledgment for my Advice and Services. But rather than accept the paultry Recompence of half a Guinea,—when my Services richly deserv'd a whole one,—I gave her the Bit of Gold back again, and told her, I wou'd make her a Present of the Cure. Not but that,

had

had ſhe offer'd me a Guinea,—it might, perhaps, have prevailed upon my Modeſty, to give it a gracious Acceptance. Now poſſibly this young Woman might (in the ſecret Receſſes of her Heart) ſay of me, upon this Occaſion,—as it was ſaid of *Martin Luther*——in the famous Bull of his Anathematization;—and there we find, that, after his Holineſs (who then ſate in the pontificial Chair) had branded, and ſtigmatized honeſt *Martin* with all the odious Vices, Depravities and Corruptions that human Nature is capable of,—he ſums up all; by ſaying, *Immo*; *Bellua contemnit Aurum.* Neverthelefs, the beſt Commentators, in their Expoſitions and Interpretations upon this Article, do hold, and maintain, that *Martin* knew the Value (both the abſolute and comparative) of Metals, as well as any one of them all;—and ſo in Truth do I.——But (be it here known and underſtood) that apoſtate, perfidious, treacherous, inſidious, iniquitous, and pernicious Son of the holy apoſtolick Church (*Martin Luther* by Name) having long and obſtinately withſtood (*Firſt*) the Perſuaſions and Entreaties; and (*Secondly*) the Threats and Menaces of the Holy See:—So when, at length, mighty Bribes were offerd him, (ſuch Bribes as wou'd preponderate the Virtue and Fortitude of any one now-a-days)—*Martin* (who was a very wiſe Man) judg'd it was then too late;—that it was altogether inconſiſtent with his Honour and with his Conſiſtency of Conduct, which he affected to ſupport, to accept of them.—And upon ſuch his Refuſal of the good and gracious Offers that were made to *Martin*, the then *Pope* (that Seat and Source of infallible Perfection, Wiſdom and Righteouſneſs) quite miſtaking the true Motives of *Martin's* Conduct, imputed

puted that to a beastly sordid Nature,—which was, in reality (or at least affectedly) the Effect of pure Virtue and Fortitude;—and such as few—very few—are now-a-days possess'd of:—But so much for a Digression; which tho' somewhat long, has the Merit to plead that it is much in the modern Taste.—— Now to return to the Case,—one wou'd naturally think, and conclude, that my signal Success in treating it, together with my very generous disinterested Behaviour, shou'd have engaged, and secured to me (*in perpetuitatem*) a Preference (in the Estimation and Opinion of that Family) to all other Physicians whatever. But whosoever may infer and conclude so, will be much mistaken in their Calculations:——For I have never since received any one Instance of Friendship, Favour, or Good-will, from that Family, nor from any of their Adherents.

NOTWITHSTANDING I have met with this very ungracious, unworthy Treatment from many Persons in this Country,—(but those, perhaps, none of the most clear sighted and discerning) yet I flatter myself with the Hopes that my Comportment has always been such as specified the Gentleman, the Man of Honour, and the Man of Probity and Integrity.—And, indeed, the Time has been (unless I am much misinformed) when I have been consider'd, by many Persons hereabouts, as a peculiar Blessing to the Country,—on Account, I suppose, of the chearful and ready Assistance I always gave to the Poor and Needy,—as well as, perhaps, on Account of the many Cures I have perform'd, upon Persons in a different Sphere, in very intricate arduous Cases.——But it seems now as if all my past Atchievements were quite cancell'd cell'd, and obliterated,—and I was ſunk into utter Oblivion.

But further,—ſuppoſe, even, that I had had no Experience in this Country—or the Country had had no Experience of me,—that is—ſuppoſing I had not performed one ſingle Cure ſince I have been here—yet one wou'd imagine that the many Works which I have penn'd and publiſh'd —and I have done as much that Way as moſt of the Faculty—all of which have been well receiv-ed; and ſome of them much applauded by the more candid and judicious Part of our Phyſicians: —Theſe Things one wou'd imagine might be ſufficient to ſpecify of me and teſtify for me; but —*Populus vult decipi—Et, ſi vult deſcipi, deſcipiatur.* This Indeed has been the Characteriſtic of the Plebs, as well as of People in general, of groſs heavy Intellects in all Ages,—theſe Folks will be deceiv'd and gull'd,—they will run, with the utmoſt avidity and ſpeed, after the very Name of a Doctor,—ſuppoſe the Man who ſupports it, has no more Senſe than a Gooſe—or no more Brains than a Hobbyhorſe.—And hence it is, that we ſee Dr. *Ward* and Dr. *Rock* ride triumphant thro' the Streets,—whilſt many Phyſicians of great Ingenuity and Merit are buried in Obſcurity.

But notwithſtanding this general Defection of the People and the conſequent Deſertion of Practice which I have ſuffer'd from it—(yet, for ſuch is my Conſtitution and Temperament) I have always look'd upon theſe Things, and reflected upon them in a manner becoming a Philoſopher. And I hope I have behaved under my adverſe Fortune, with as much Equanimity as any other Perſon cou'd or wou'd have done,—and that I think, is making the best of a bad Market.

I HAVE, in good Truth, been so far from feeling any Chagrin, or Dejection of Spirits from it, that I have been in all Companies, just as gay and merry, as if I was in the Zenith of Fame, Practice and Renown,—even as much as if I was the primary medical Idol in all the Country.——This, perhaps, may be admitted as a presumptive Proof that I possess some Tincture of heroic Virtue—— *Namque Arduis præcipue emicat Virtus.*——Nevertheless (I must own it) ever since the 17th of *March*, when those Secrets were communicated to me, my Indignation and Resentment have been raised to a very high Pitch indeed,—and very sufficient Reason I think I had for it.——If I shou'd return into this Country; (which is not improbable) and shou'd resolve to continue in it; I may, possibly, (in case what I have already said is not effectual) use some further and future Endeavours to convince the People of their Errors and Mistakes—I will not be wanting in the Exertion of proper Endeavours, to turn the Comforts of a fine Cure into Profit and Emolument.

I HOPE (and perhaps am not mistaken) that I have the good and laudable Dispositions of Friendship, Generosity, Benevolence, Beneficence, Hospitality and Charity, as deeply imprinted in my Nature as any Man living. If I was conscious that I had not—I wou'd endeavour to cultivate and improve them.——However, this has been, heretofore, my peculiar Characteristic; and this Tribute of Praise has been often paid to me, and hence it seems to me the more surprizing and amazing that I should be thus slandered and scandalized.—Indeed I am not a little surprized and astonished at their Impudence, in presuming it,—as it must, I think, be imagined that I am always able to defend myself, and to refute their impious villainous Slanders.

It wou'd, perhaps, appear strange and amazing to the more learned and judicious Part of the World, (*i. e.* to publick Universities, both at Home and Abroad,—— by many of which my Works have been received and esteemed) shou'd they chance to hear that my Conduct in Practice has met with so much Censure and Blame.

It has long since been a Custom with me, at my leisure Hours, to exercise my Mind (in order to improve and enrich it) in almost every Branch of Science;—and hence (besides the many Works which I have exhibited to the Publick) I have amused and entertain'd myself in Writing,—not only on Physic,—strictly speaking,—but likewise on Physics, Ethics, Metaphysics, Mathematics, Law, and Divinity,—or more properly—Theology.——But after all, it seems as if no Virtues, no Accomplishments, nor any Atchievements of mine were to be had in Regard or Remembrance; —— but I must, at all Events, (cost what it will,) be persecuted, run down, and earthed.—There are some Persons of the Pharmacential Order in this Country—whom I cannot, in my private Judgment, hold altogether guiltless.—There are particularly two of these Gentlemen (that live in Market Towns, at some Miles distance) who most zealously and officiously recommend another Physician, in Preference to, and

in

in Prejudice of me. And this, I dare ſay, they do (one of them more eſpecially) againſt their own better Judgment;—and in and by this Conduct, as I apprehend, they expoſe either their own Underſtanding, or elſe their Honeſty and Probity, as well as Conſcience, to juſt Cenſure and Reproach.

I CAN'T help thinking (tho' I may, perhaps, be miſtaken) that theſe Gentlemen are obliged, in Honour and Conſcience (when they know there is a Phyſician in the Neighbourhood of ſuperior Judgment and Skill,—— and one who may be had with equal Conveniency in all Reſpects) to propoſe him at leaſt; not but that the good People (the Patients) have, after all, an undoubted Right to die, and be d—n'd in their own Way.

I HAVE heard ſome of theſe Gentlemen (occaſionally) reply very gravely, that they always left it to their Patients to chuſe what Phyſician they pleas'd.—— But even this (ſuppoſing it to be true, which I do not) is perhaps a criminal Omiſſion; 'tis a Thing well known, to ſuch as are acquainted with the World, that, in the Medical Sphere eſpecially, errant Blockheads ſhall, ſometimes, (either by Chance or perſonal Favour) ſtep into great Fame and Practice,——whilſt ſome other Phyſicians, of incomparably greater Sagacity and Skill, ſhall be utterly neglected and buried in Oblivion.

I, MYSELF, have known this Obſervation verified in many Inſtances,—and ſuch extraordinary Phænomena as theſe do appear in the World, every Day almoſt; tho' the undiſcerning Part of Mankind

kind don't perceive it.——These Things intimate, or rather specify, either the Imbecility of the human Judgment, or else the Pravity and Corruption of our Morals.——I have been well informed, and assured, that some Years ago, even in our famous University of *Oxford*, a certain Physician (now dead) was very zealously patronized, and strenuously push'd into Practice, (without the least Shadow of Merit, in him, to authorize and countenance it.) And this by the greatest Man of the Faculty in *Oxford*, or perhaps, in the whole Nation.——And all this was done (as 'tis shrewdly suspected) in mere Opposition to another Physician who, is confessedly one of as bright a Genius as most of the Age and Faculty.

I AM well informed, and assured, that the Gentleman I allude to (in Opposition to whom this Farce was Acted) is a Person of a very bright aspiring Genius,—and has natural Endowments superior to most,—tho' I think it is generally allow'd that he has not endeavour'd so much as cou'd be wish'd, to cultivate and enrich his natural Gifts and Endowments, by an assiduous Application to Study;—so I think this Gentleman seems to emulate, if not to equal, the late great Doctor *Ratcliff*,—of whom a similar Character is at this Day given.—But tho' this Gentleman (who is at this Time a Practitioner at *Oxford*) does not apply himself so rigorously to Study, as these of a saturnine Complexion must necessarily do, if they wou'd make any Figure in Life; yet he is, by all, allow'd to be a very great Physician,—as well in the practical Part, as in the Speculative. He is generally allow'd to be a Man of a very quick Penetration; and of great Sagacity and Judgment also;

—and

—and ſuch happy natural Gifts as theſe will always (my Word for it) preponderate and triumph over the heavy Fruits and Effects of laborious Study—unaſſiſted by a bright Genius.—In fine—this Gentleman (according to the general Character I have receiv'd of him) ſeems to have all the Seeds of Medicine, (*i. e.* all the natural neceſſary Requiſites proper to form a great Phyſician) innate and inherent in him. So that we may very juſtly compare him to the Stone in Pyrrhus's Ring,—which, as 'tis ſaid, had *Apollo* and the Nine *Muſes* interwoven in the Veins of it by Nature: This Gentleman will reflect a Luſture on the Name of *Pitt*,—as well as an Honour on the Place of his Birth,——which as I am told is in this County.

'Tis a Thing much to be deplored, that in a wiſe, good, and well regulated Government, ſuch as ours confeſſedly is, the Superintendance and Care of People's Lives and Healths ſhould not be more confin'd, and better ſecur'd to them;—and this, by limiting the Exerciſe of the Medical Art or Science, to ſuch only as had manifeſted ſuperior Endowments and Accompliſhments,—as well natural as acquired;—and if proper Cenſors were appointed by the Legiſlature—capable to diſcern, and ingenious enough to confeſs and declare——who were fit, and who not fit, to be truſted in ſuch momentous Concerns;—and that, in Conſequence of it, the Body Politic of Phyſick was to be ****** of all its uſeleſs deſtructive Members—I Queſtion much if (under a Reciſion of one Half or two Thirds of the preſent Number) the Public wou'd not be much better ſecured, by thoſe that remained, of their Lives and Healths.

After I had finished the above Narration (which makes the last, tho' not the least Part of the whole Work) and had maturely perused, weighed, and considered it,—I can't help owning that I thought it consistent with Prudence and good Policy not to publish it, as it may possibly alienate from me the Friendship and Good-will of many Persons I am acquainted with.—And, in Truth, upon the first springing up of these Suggestions, and Scruples, I was much inclin'd, and almost resolv'd, to suppress it.——But then (whilst I was deliberating upon it, and not yet determined) the just Indignation and Resentment which I had conceived and harboured, against the forementioned base Slanders and Calumnies;——these Things rose in Judgment against my pacific Disposition, and they peremptorily demanded that I should offer this Sacrifice to them, in order to appease, in some Measure, their Anger——even tho' it was at the manifest Risque of forfeiting half the Friends I have in these Parts. In fine—the Demands and Clamours of those Passions were so raging and impetuous, that they even forced me to comply, and gratify them—and in the Conclusion—I thought it was, of the two, better and more eligible to risque the Forfeiture of all the Friends I have in these Parts, rather than lie under so false, so base, and villainous an Imputation.

My Way and Rule of acting is, and has been, to make myself known to, and acquainted with all such Persons as I think worthy of it—and this as soon as possible—but, when once I perceive that any of those with whom I have commenced and cultivated an Acquaintance, apostatize and go a whoring after other Idols, (not that I count myself one of the

Num-

Number) I gradually decline, and at length quite drop their Acquaintance.

I OBSERVED by our Weekly Journal of the 28th of *April*, that a Gentleman, who was my good Acquaintance, and my profeſs'd Friend, is gone to the *Elyſian* Shades. Now, as this Gentleman had always profeſs'd a great Friendſhip for me, and had intimated, that, upon Occaſion, I ſhould be his Phyſician, ſo muſt neceſſarily judge and conclude that his Opinion of me had been poiſoned and perverted by the above-mentioned ſlanderous Reports. But if I am ſurprized and amazed at the Alienation of that Gentleman's good Opinion of me,—I am no leſs ſo to find that his Phyſician (whoever he was) ſhould let him languiſh ſo long; and, in the End, die—without deſiring ſome other Phyſicians's Aſſiſtance in Conſultation:—But, perhaps, the Phyſician concern'd might think (as I dare ſay the grand Monarch *Lewis* XIV. of *France*, would have thought upon the like Occaſion) *viz.* that his deſiring another Phyſician's Aſſiſtance would be a manifeſt Diminution of his own Preeminence; but we (who know ſomething of the World, and can dive into the ſecret Receſſes of People's Hearts) ſee plainly and clearly that ſome of the Brethren (even of the ſacred Miſſion of Phyſic) are ſo much attached to the firſt Perſon, as never to regard the Second or the Third: And, in Conſequence of ſuch a perſonal Attachment, I dare ſay, many a poor Patient dies,—who might otherwiſe have been recover'd.

I (for my Part) am always ready and willing to have Aſſiſtance in all Caſes which appear very dangerous: And as I have done this in ſeveral Inſtances,

ſo

so I have had Opportunities and Occasions of making (some pretty severe) but very just Criticisms, in my private Judgment, upon my Colleagues. And I may, I think, suppose that all such Persons, of good Understanding and Judgment, as know me, in my Fruits and Effects, will allow me to be a tolerable good Critic in Things physical and philosophical. And perhaps they will allow that I may now and then (without Offence to Modesty, and without the Imputation of Arrogance) presume to criticize upon the Brethren.—I have (I own it) been often induced (when I have heard the crude Notions of some of my Brethren) to think and to say, (if alas! Learning, Reading, and Study, tend no further than this) why then it may, at this Time, be most righteously said of Physic, as it has heretofore been most impiously said of Christianity, that verily it is not mysterious.

The Publication of this Piece having been (much against my Inclinations) postponed for several Weeks.—This Interval of Time has proved to me that my Predictions (as to the rapid Progress and Fortune of Inoculation) are abundantly fulfilled;—which I am extreamly well pleased with.

Now, the Reader is desired to excuse some Inaccuracies of Style—which are but too palpable and visible.—Both Parts of the Work, but especially the last and largest Part, were wrote in the greatest Hurry. And the last Part, particularly, when my Mind and Thoughts were ruffled and confused to a very great Degree, by hearing of those base slanderous Reports,

P. S. Having just now the *Gentleman's Magazine* for last Month under my Inspection, I there find (*p.* 126) a Piece which suggests some Objections to, or Doubts concerning the Practice of Inoculation —— upon which (lest it should shake the Faith of weak, irresolute Minds, and tend to the Prejudice of Inoculation) I shall make some Remarks by Way of Prevention. The first Objection or Doubt is, whether such Persons as have received the Small Pox by Inoculation, are absolutely secured from having it again in the natural Way.— And whether this Disease given by Inoculation, may not prove fatal.—The first Part of this complicated Doubt may appeal to, and rely upon, the universal Consent and Suffrage of Mankind—which attests, that a Person who has had the Small Pox by Inoculation, is not susceptible of it, or liable to it, any more. But the least Part of that Doubt is not intitled to so positive and peremptory an Answer: For, according to the general Opinion and Reports that at present obtain—this same Practice, tho' comparatively, and that in a high Degree safe and salutary, is not absolutely void of Danger:—— For we may gather, from general Accounts of the Matter, that about one in 130 dies of the Small Pox by Inoculation.

The other Doubt or Scruple, which is of a more religious Cast, is concerning the Extent of the parental Authority over their Children.——He apprehends, that Parents (by Virtue of this Authority) have not a Right to inflict a Disease on their Children (how light soever the Disease, and how small soever the Danger may be) when they are not of Years and Understanding sufficient to determine for themselves: And he imagines, that should a Child,

whom

whom its Parents had caused to be inoculated, di of the Small Pox, the Laws both of God and Society would call the Parents in Question for it. *i, e.* (as he must mean) put them to Death for it.

Then the Author (in order to justify and fortify his Scruples) supposes a Case as a Parallel to it. If a Man (says he, should put a Sum of Money (suppose 100 or 1000 *l.*) into a Lottery, which Sum had been given to his Child by a Relation, and the Money should be all lost by the Bargain——the Parent, in that Case, would be obliged, by a Court of Equity, to make the Money good to his Child.——Upon this I have to observe——That if a Parent puts a Sum of Money, which was given or bequeathed to his Child by some Relation into a Lottery, or shall place it out upon a precarious Security, on Condition of an exorbitant Interest for it,—with Intent to take and apply all the Profits and Advantages arising from it to his own proper Use:——In that Case, indeed, the Man wou'd be oblig'd (*Fore Conscientiæ, Foro Rationis, atque Foro judicii*) to make the Money with legal Interest good to his Child—in Case the Money shou'd be lost. Because no Man is authorized to sport and play with another's Property, (not even his own Child's) with a View to his own Profit and Advantage, but he must stand to the Risk of it, if lost. But let us suppose the contrary of this,—and that it be made appear, upon good Evidence, that the Father was a discreet, indulgent and affectionate Parent; and that he manifestly acted upon a very probable and warrantable Scheme, for the good of his Child—or in that View at least; I am very much of Opinion that, in such a Case, the Court of Equity wou'd wou'd acquit him;—tho' perhaps a Court of Common Law might decree againſt him.—But in good Truth, I take the Parallel itſelf to be very imperfect, jejune and trifling—For there is very little Parity in the Caſes,—every Parent is oblig'd by the Laws of God, of Nature, and Society, to take Care of his Children.—Thoſe very Laws direct and inſtruct us to provide, by all proper Care and Cautions, not only for their Preſervation and Health, but for their future Comfort and Happineſs alſo——And therefore the ſubjecting a Child to a ſlight (tho' preſent and certain) Inconveniency; in order to free it, and ſecure it, from and againſt the Dread and Fear of catching a Diſtemper that may prove fatal:—This is altogether conſiſtent with parental Affection and Authority;—with ſtrict Prudence, and good Oeconomy.

F I N I S.

E R R A T A.

PAge 4. Line 9. *for* Mingretians *read* Mingrelians. Line 20, and 23, of ſame Page *f* Opperation *r*. Operation —Page 5. Line 16. *f.* reaſonable *r* rational. Line 28 of the ſame Page, *r. it is not univerſally ſubſcribed to* Page 8. Line 10. *f.* ganty *r*. gouty. Line 17, and 18, of ſame Page, *f.* morbic *r*. morbid. Line 29. ſame Page, *r. Laudatur ab his—Culpatur ab illis.* In the laſt Line, *f.* ample *r*. amiable.

CPSIA information can be obtained at www.ICGtesting.com
Printed in the USA
BVOW08s1115031114

373436BV00015B/431/P